Opioids

In Chronic Pain Management

A Guide for Patients

This book expresses the views of J. Kimber Rotchford, M.D., a pain management and addiction medicine specialist. The book is published by Olympas Medical Services, Ltd. of Port Townsend, Washington.

Printed in The United States of America

First Edition 2017
Second Edition 2018

Cover Art is reproduced from the private collection of the author.
Front Cover: *Nice to Meet You, Mr. Crow* by artist Gilchun Koh
Back Cover: *James K Dragon* by Maggie Roe

ISBN-13: 978-1984377975
ISBN-10: 1984377973

Contact the Publisher
Olympas Medical Services
J. Kimber Rotchford, M.D.
1136 Water St. Suite 107
Port Townsend, WA 98368

www.OPAS.us
staff@OPAS.us
This book can be ordered from Amazon and retail stores
Purchasers of this book are invited to download a PDF copy with clickable links at:
DrRotchford.com/guide

Opioids

In Chronic Pain Management

A Guide for Patients

by

J. Kimber Rotchford, M.D., M.P.H.

TABLE OF CONTENTS

Foreword by the Author

Pain and suffering are ubiquitous. No quick answer explains why pain and suffering exist. Indeed, entire religions have been built on how best to address suffering. This guide does not pretend to explain suffering nor how to eliminate it. It intends to help patients better appreciate the risks and benefits of using opioids in chronic pain management. The guide introduces principles, alternatives, and adjunctive treatments, which are often effective in better managing chronic pain.

No clear biomarkers are available to help physicians determine when to prescribe opioids for chronic pain. We depend on a patient's history and other contextual variables to help evaluate the need for opioids. Fortunately, studies of select populations and evidence-based findings do provide some help in predicting which patients with chronic pain are likely to respond favorably to opioids.

Prescribing opioids for chronic pain is similar to prescribing insulin for diabetes. Dosing and indications are best individualized. By measuring blood sugars, we know how much insulin to prescribe for a diabetic. Through current measures of pain levels and functioning, we have guides to help us predict proper dosing of opioids. In both cases, follow up and professional monitoring are essential for the best outcomes. For select patients, opioids save lives and limit serious disability. As with insulin, one does not want to prescribe opioids, when they might be of limited benefit or when opioids could have undue risks or complications, particularly as compared to other possible interventions. Culturally, we are inclined to focus on the risks of chronic opioid use. Frequently overlooked, however, when managing chronic pain, as with diabetes, are the complications of under-treatment. Poorly managed pain can be seriously disabling and even life-threatening.

Simple *yes* or *no* answers are commonly sought. In answering the question of when to use opioids for chronic pain management, the best response is: It depends! For a new patient seeking pain management, I outline pertinent considerations that help us judge when the risks and benefits of using opioids justify their use in chronic pain management. Individualized medical care is always best. And while the best care for an individual is often supported by population studies, which evaluate similar patients, the astute clinician always tailors care to the individual. Medicine most often involves educated gambling and it helps to know the odds prior to placing a bet. Once the bet is placed, it is essential to determine if it is paying off or whether another bet could be even more helpful. This guide is intended, with the help of professional oversight, to help patients better appreciate the odds, bets, and payoffs of opioid use in the management of chronic pain.

J. Kimber Rotchford, M.D.

From the Editor

Dr. Rotchford is acknowledged by his community as a caring and compassionate physician. In 2009, he was the honored recipient of the Heart of Service award sponsored by local newspapers and local Rotary clubs. As a researcher, a voracious reader, and a prolific writer, Dr. Rotchford strives to stay current with the latest discoveries in the medical and social sciences. His fluency in current understandings is reflected in his publications, essays, and handouts related to pain management and substance abuse. His expertise in Public Health has also prompted him to write multiple papers on the social and Public Health implications of opioid use and abuse.

This book, *Opioids in Chronic Pain Management – A Guide for Patients*, is part of a series of publications which promote access to Dr. Rotchford's expertise in helping patients with chronic pain and substance use disorders.

Dan Youra, Editor

Introduction

Introduction

This guide is primarily for patients with chronic pain who are asking whether the use of opioids is helpful or not. A long time ago, the Greeks recognized that "one person's food is another's poison." Evidence-based modern medicine is built upon the study of populations or groups of patients. Clinical evidence in conjunction with basic scientific understandings guide clinicians to better care for a patient. While population studies are most useful, as already stressed in the forward, the best medical care is individualized.

As is the case with any potent prescription, a patient is wise to seek professional advice before a medication is used. Historically, physicians are the experts in prescribing opioids. Their prescribing authority as it pertains to opioids has been significantly compromised within the United States. The explanations for this are likely to be debated for they are complex and challenge many fixed beliefs within the American culture.

Within the United States government regulators and third-party payers (insurance companies, Medicare, Medicaid) have become the default authorities regarding the proper use of opioids. Regulators decide appropriate diagnoses and sometimes limit certain opioids to specific settings or prescribers. They now determine the nature of care, oversight, doses, access, etc. Based on payments, third-party payers commonly judge which opioid and how much of an opioid is appropriate. Despite the concerns about financial conflicts of interest, third-parties have been emboldened to judge what constitutes safe prescribing. The involvement by third parties and regulators, for better and for ill, compromises physician discretion and professional care.

Rules and regulations regarding potentially life-threatening substances are useful. As with opioids themselves, too much or too little regulation is sometimes a challenge to judge. Regarding the current opioid misuse crisis, potential explanations and solutions are provided in another publication, *Opidemic* [23].

When it comes to prescribing opioids, physicians have become understandably fearful. The United States Attorney General in 2017 overtly threatened prescribers with serious legal consequences for alleged inappropriate prescribing of opioids. The underlying assumption is that regulators and others are well suited to determine what constitutes appropriate prescribing.

Physicians' fears are justified. Is it safe for them to prescribe? The prescribing of opioids for chronic pain in the United States appears to have become more a matter of law and politics than one of proper medical care based on a patient's specific needs.

Even well-trained and well-intentioned experts in pain management and addiction medicine can come under serious attack. Regulatory investigations and criminal charges have serious repercussions to careers and to patients cared for. Physicians can be investigated, harassed, and even lose their licenses. This has happened even in cases where patient outcomes were arguably quite good.

Perhaps a physician outside the protection of a large institution can no longer find it prudent or reasonable to prescribe long-term opioids? Given the regulatory and third-party pressures, many physicians choose not to prescribe opioids for chronic conditions, even when patients would surely benefit. This is grievous.

Most physicians are well trained to prescribe opioids in the context of acute pain, defined as pain which lasts less than a month or so. When it comes to managing chronic pain and opioid use disorders, there is a widespread need for education, even among seasoned and otherwise capable physicians. The majority of physicians do not commonly diagnose opioid use disorders and even fewer are familiar with the formal criteria. This remains true despite evidence that 20-25% of patients on chronic opioid agonist therapy (COAT) for pain have a significant opioid use disorder (addiction). Agonist therapy refers to pain pills and substances that stimulate the opioid (mu) receptors in the brain.

Many physicians continue to explain chronic pain based on standard diagnoses that imply tissue damage as the primary cause of the pain. While this explanation is typically true with acute pain, it becomes the exception with chronic pain. Western science has confirmed that the central nervous system involvement is of primary importance in chronic pain. That is to say central nervous system dysfunction is the rule in most cases of chronic pain. Support for the central nervous system is always useful in chronic pain management. While nociception (tissue damage) is stressful and may interfere with healthy functioning of the central nervous system, limiting nociception is rarely enough in managing chronic complex pain. This is in contrast to the treatment of acute pain when procedures and surgical interventions often help. This is also in contrast to when chronic pain exists and surgical procedures and "acute" medicinal interventions may make matters worse.

With chronic pain the central nervous system adapts to the painful input, and there are corresponding neuroadaptations (changes in neural circuits). Sleep deprivation, mood disorders, and other stressors to brain health, even when there is no apparent source of peripheral nociception (tissue damage), all contribute to serious and sometimes widespread pain.

Opioids are prescribed to help the body and central nervous system work better. The ways opioids help some brains function better and limit pain are complex and not entirely understood. In metaphorical terms, opioids turn down the volume on pain "noise." In addition, opioids are potent, anti-anxiety medications. Throughout modern times they have been used as mood enhancers and, to a lesser degree, mood stabilizers.

Bottom line, opioids when prescribed appropriately are most often therapeutic and can be life saving. They, like all potent medications, can be misused and present lethal consequences. It makes sense to have opioids prescribed by a knowledgeable clinician, and for them to be used only as prescribed.

This guide is designed to empower patients and their advocates to obtain proper pain management, with or without opioids. As already mentioned, opioids can be part of a healthy solution, or they can contribute to poor pain management, other complications, and even an early death.

This guide starts with a brief review of the discussions commonly provided to a new patient during their initial pain management consultation. Given the specialized nature of the author's practice, these new patient consultations commonly hinge upon whether opioids are part of the problem or part of a solution.

Chapter One

Initial Consultation—Opioids in Chronic Pain Management

Chapter One

Initial Consultation — Opioids in Chronic Pain Management

This chapter focuses on the initial consultation. The five components of the initial consultation are:

1. Assess current pain levels and function.

2. Introduce patients to the notion that chronic pain is different than acute pain (it feels the same as acute pain and may or may not limit function in similar ways).

3. Determine whether opioids are part of the solution or part of the problem.

4. Assess other interventions or support, in addition to or besides opioids, which could better help manage the pain.

5. Establish an initial plan for clinical progress in pain management.

1. Assess Current Pain Levels and Function

Questionnaires and other clinical tools help determine the need for and success of pain management. Some questionnaires are designed to evaluate pain and disability related to specific types of pain such as low back pain. Most physicians have access to these instruments, and they are often quite helpful. We use a customized version of the Wisconsin

Brief Pain Inventory. A score of 100 is associated with the maximum amount of possible pain and pain-related dysfunction during the past week. (See Appendix 2)

The responses to the different questions are subjective. One patient's "five" might be another's "seven" or "eight," or vice versa. Nonetheless, these questionnaires allow a valid and reliable comparison of scores between patients and allow us to observe and validate individualized progress over time. Pain, like blood pressure and other physiological processes, varies over time. A specific score, by itself, has limited value. Changes in pain scores, observed over time, is what matters.

Appendix 2, at the end, includes a copy of the Global Pain Questionnaire & Brief Follow-up Inventory. The Brief Follow-up Inventory, or BFU, evaluates overall brain health and recovery. Poorly managed chronic pain implies that the brain is not working as well as it could. While the BFU Inventory has not been formally validated, it has been found to be helpful in assessing overall progress. At the least, the BFU Inventory gives patients another opportunity to determine their progress or lack thereof.

2. Chronic Pain vs. Acute Pain

Chronic pain and acute pain are concepts introduced earlier in this guide. The differences between the two types of pain are important to recognize. This can be challenging because, while the differences are important, their similarities are apparent.

Acute pain is "new" pain and is often associated with some tissue damage. While growing up, children commonly experience forms of acute pain. Knees are scraped and noggins are bruised. Cuts and insect bites cause pain. Hence, as one gets older, one may assume that all pain is related to "tissue damage."

It should not though be assumed that all pain is best managed like acute pain. A hug, a dressing, a suture, or at least a bandaid is what one might expect to help with acute pain. Perhaps the child or young adult was given an over the counter pain pill? Our early experiences condition us to believe that a pain pill is often an effective way to address pain, whether acute or chronic.

For more severe forms of pain, whether from serious injuries or surgical procedures, one may have been exposed to opioids. As previously noted, when we experience pain as adults, it makes sense we would look for similar explanations and remedies which worked in the past.

In contrast with acute pain, the severity of chronic pain does not correlate well with peripheral tissue damage or dysfunction. In general, chronic pain often does not respond well to acute pain remedies. When one sees a freshly broken bone on X-ray, it readily explains the reason for the pain. With chronic pain, however, there is a poor correlation between the amount of pain a patient is experiencing and diagnostic X-rays and even more refined imaging techniques. For example, take the case of chronic pain associated with degenerative arthritis (osteoarthritis or "bad joints"). Some patients have minor or no pain even when there are serious X-ray findings of degenerative arthritis. Conversely, horrible pain may be associated with only limited changes in the joint or other structures.

Levels of inflammation and other local factors, not readily appreciated by standard imaging techniques, can play a role in contributing to the pain associated with chronic, complex pain. Inevitably though, in addition to local factors, one is dealing with neural dysfunction, whether in the periphery or in the central nervous system.

References online and elsewhere review the importance of treating chronic pain different than acute pain[1-5]. We now consider chronic pain as a disease, in and of itself, with significant and objective findings of inflammation and dysfunction in the brain, spinal cord, and occasionally the autonomic nervous system. Neuropathy related chronic pain is a relatively unique form of chronic pain and often benefits from specific remedies in addition to those typically used with chronic pain. [5,6].

3. Are Opioids Part the Problem?

This is often the most "charged" part of an initial consultation. Most patients, both those referred by a colleague and those who independently seek out specialized care, are concerned about the need for opioids to manage their painful conditions.

Because of the differences between chronic and acute pain, it can still surprise many colleagues when opioids are part of a solution, and often essentially so. The most common reason for opioids being a clear part of the solution is when a patient has a significant opioid use disorder. Most frequently, this disorder stems from long-standing exposure to prescribed opioids. In a small number of cases, the opioid use disorder developed independently by means of illicit opioid abuse, such as with heroin or "street" pain pills.

An opioid use disorder implies the brain has been changed, most often permanently, as a result of being exposed to opioids. In a published paper on "Chronic Opioid Agonist Therapy" (COAT)[7], the author estimates that about 20% of patients who receive opioids chronically for pain develop a significant opioid use disorder. Recently, estimates from the Centers for Disease Control (CDC) are as high as 25% of patients on COAT develop an opioid use disorder. The criteria for an opioid use disorder or opiate dependence can be found readily.[8] The criteria represent the conclusions of experts and the leading research regarding the best predictors of who has an opioid use disorder. None of the criteria have anything to do with moral or even legal concerns. The criteria are such that it becomes relatively easy to establish or exclude the diagnosis. It remains to the astute clinician to establish the severity of the disease. See Appendix 1, at the end, for a brief screening questionnaire related to opioid use disorders.

As of now, there are no established biomarkers for an opioid use disorder, as for diabetes and many other chronic relapsing diseases. While there is quite a bit of ignorance as to the criteria, even among physicians, they are the best we have. The criteria remain primarily dependent on an accurate and thorough history taking. Occasionally, a physical exam or laboratory finding helps alert the clinician to the possibility or likelihood of a patient having the disease. As already stated, Appendix One contains a valid and reliable questionnaire that allows a physician to readily predict whether a patient has an opioid use disorder (OUD).

Twenty to twenty-five percent of patients who develop an opioid use disorder (addiction) have risk factors. Genetics play a large role. Another important factor is the age when one is first exposed to significant amounts of opioids. The earlier the age, the greater the risk. Exposure prior to brain maturity is particularly risky. We also know that significant trauma in the past, whether physical, sexual, psychological, or even spiritual, greatly increases risks. Comorbid substance use disorders, whether legal or not, such as alcohol and tobacco use disorders, are major risk factors. Other comorbid mental health problems increase the risks of an OUD.

Based on the patient's history, familiarity with the formal criteria, as well as the risk factors, a diagnosis of an opioid use disorder can generally be readily made. In less clear cases, the best course of action is to be conservative and to treat patients as though they have an opioid use disorder, because when left untreated the prognosis is poor. A conservative approach is particularly true when the patient's risk factors are significant. This approach is similar to an emergency room physician treating someone with chest pain as though they are having a heart attack until established otherwise.

In brief, if a patient has an opioid use disorder, particularly if moderate or severe, the prognosis is poor without ongoing agonist (opioid) therapy. The literature and expert consensus confirming this are significant[9-11] compared to common indications for other medical care, such as blood pressure lowering. The prognosis is predictably poor with abstinence-based approaches when a patient has comorbid serious pain or other mental health disorders.

There are perhaps 30% of patients on COAT who expectedly will do better if tapered off opioids. These patients have been "neuro-sensitized" to opioids and, as a result of long-term use of opioids, their pain thresholds become quite low. We know this from animal studies and clinical observations confirm. While their pain might seem to be better as the result of taking a pill, as a matter of neuroadaptations, continued use of opioids is making pain worse.

The problem is trying to sort out which patients fit into this category. There are some possible clinical indicators based on history and findings, but generally the only way to know is a trial where the patient is slowly tapered off of opioids and is closely followed.

How about the other 50% or so of patients who are on COAT? Are the opioids part of the solution or part of the problem? Sometimes the clinical history tells the story. If a patient has taken opioids for years, perhaps is elderly, and has done well with opioids with little or no side effects, and is apparently otherwise healthy, this sort of history supports ongoing, judicious use of opioids. In the author's opinion, despite extra risks associated with sedatives and opioids in the elderly, older patients who are functioning well on opioids with limited side-effects are best not be put at risk from unnecessary withdrawal or unmitigated pain.

Clinical context needs to be judiciously reviewed to best assess who is to be tapered off opioids and how quickly. Some patients, even those with an opioid use disorder, want to be immediately tapered off opioids. Understandably, for who would want to have to take a medication to remain functional, especially a medication with all of the social concerns and current stigma associated with its use? In those cases, when unable to establish the diagnosis of a significant opioid use disorder, and there is a lack of serious or multiple risk factors, an attempt to gently taper a patient off opioids is surely warranted. Meanwhile, the patient needs assistance to find other ways to assure pain is well managed. As already stated, routine and regular follow-up is indicated to assure progress with pain management and overall health.

There is much to be written on the subject of whether opioids are part of the problem or part of the solution. In this brief discussion, I have not explored the social and community risks associated with prescribing opioids. The focus here remains on patient health. That being said, healthy patients generally make for healthy communities.

Lastly, for those patients who will likely benefit from chronic opioid agonist therapy (COAT), the use of long-acting forms of opioids is most often advised. The brain benefits from staying in a relative state of homeostasis. This simply means that the brain doesn't like its internal environment to change. Short-acting opiates, as appropriate as they are for acute pain, play a limited role in managing chronic, complex pain. Short-acting opioids for chronic pain are indicated and can be quite useful when there are acute flares of an underlying disease such as rheumatoid arthritis or gout. An essential intention of effective chronic pain management is to help the brain and the rest of the central nervous system function as well as possible.

4. What Other Ways Might Improve Central Nervous System Function and Help with Pain Management?

In addition to opioids, many other ways are available to better manage pain. Unfortunately, it is commonplace to encounter problems with access and availability of effective alternatives. There are a myriad of approaches and ways to help brains function better. The OPAS handout, *Brain Health 101*, [12] can be helpful in regards to pain management, memory issues, and brain fog.

One of the biggest barriers to effective pain management is our relative inability to accurately predict who will respond best to which intervention. As the Greeks said long ago, "One man's food is another's poison." As a certified and longstanding member of the American Academy of Integrative Pain Management, it is clear there are many modalities which help patients to safely and effectively manage their pain. The issue often becomes: "Where does one best start?"

This question is problematic for patients, as well as for providers. We sometimes inappropriately expect patients to know what's best for them, even when we know that they are relatively uninformed and that perhaps their brains are not working properly. In addition, based on access issues related to geography and financial factors, many options are limited.

When appropriate, choices are provided and it is most often best to start with the safest options and proceed from there. The adage "First things first" works well. Let's make sure we are getting proper nutrition, exercise, and socialization to help us feel safer and less threatened. These precepts for good health are nothing new. Entire religions are built upon them.

In patients on opioids or with pain management needs, good sleep is especially important. Sleep apnea is a condition in which a patient stops breathing for short periods while sleeping. This can be highly problematic to one's overall health, let alone pain and stress levels. Sleep apnea needs to be ruled out, because opioids commonly cause or aggravate sleep apnea.

We want to make sure the body has what it needs to function properly and to be at its best. Hormone levels are to be checked. Vitamin D and other basic nutrients are to be optimized. It is useful to rule out other medical problems or substances being used that could interfere with healthy brains.

How we manage our emotions, particularly grief and anger are important in better managing pain. Many handouts and essays are available at www.OPAS.us. Several of the handouts review emotional, psychiatric, and medical concerns that contribute significantly to pain thresholds with elements of Post Traumatic Stress Disorder (PTSD) being common[13-20].

As already indicated, health is often associated with a sense of safety and well-being. Indeed, brains work best when they feel safe and are in a state of homeostasis. Situational as well as internal stresses interfere with proper brain functioning. To be healthy, over time we must attempt to eliminate internal stressors as well as external ones.

We are made to move. Movement and exercise help brains, hearts, and other organs to work better. Of course, for a number of reasons patients with chronic pain are often limited in their movements and ability to exercise. A concerted effort must be made to promote activity. Often it takes professional help with physical and occupational therapists. Professional behavioral and social support may also promote progress with movement and exercise. Yoga or Tai Qi can be life changing for some.

Co-occurring mental health conditions are common. Depression is well known to contribute to pain and can even be a primary cause. Since anxiety and Post Traumatic Stress Disorders (PTSD) are quite common, patients may benefit from treatment for these conditions.

At www.OPAS.us patients can access a myriad of ways to better manage their chronic pain. One of the biggest clinical challenges in this work is tailoring an effective program to a given patient. It is unusual for a single intervention to take care of all pain management needs. A combination of interventions are found to work best, over time.

One does not need to be free of pain in order to have a healthy and vibrant life. Indeed, an expectation to be pain free can compromise pain management. Some patients are inclined to catastrophize (imagine or foresee things as much worse than the are) when it comes to their pain. While the term "catastrophize" can be overly dramatic, it does remind us to look closely at our expectations and perceptions about what we expect to experience. Based on prior conditioning, our brains can and do play tricks on us. Magicians take advantage of this and, knowing what we are conditioned to see or experience, inevitably they are able to fool and amaze us. We are all susceptible to past conditioning. The good news is that there is overwhelming evidence that the brain can change, and all brains have what is called "neuroplasticity." This simply means we are designed to learn and heal.

The word "physician" is derived from roots which mean "teacher." A good physician promotes healing by helping bodies and brains learn healthier patterns. When one must turn for outside support or interventions, rather than depend solely on natural processes, the path is often challenging. Nonetheless, proper outside support and encouragement are often essential when it comes to managing complex chronic pain.

5. Establish an Initial Plan for Progress

Patients should always have a plan after each office visit. Using some of the basic principles already mentioned, an initial plan can readily be established, and patients are provided our "Plan Handout" (see Appendix 3). The most important part of the plan are return visits to assure progress is being made.

Another important part of the initial plan is to better ensure that a patient has an adequate health care team. No one clinician can do it all. This is particularly true when caring for more complex pain patients. Often other specialists, as well as the primary care provider, act as effective members of the team.

In summary, often the best chronic pain management is provided over time. Follow-up visits are essential, for they ensure that adequate evaluations have been made and that there is progress in pain management. This takes us to Chapter Two— Is the Plan Working?

.

Chapter Two

Is the Plan Working?

Chapter Two — Is the Plan Working?

To assess whether plans are working, follow-up visits are initially scheduled at least monthly and often on a more frequent basis. The brain generally takes at least three to six months to heal and stabilize. Not infrequently, the best results may be seen two-three years out. Fortunately, progress, or the lack thereof, often happens within weeks and months. This allows frequent follow-up visits to be helpful in monitoring progress.

A physician or patient can never be entirely sure what is going to work when it comes to managing chronic pain. The variables involved are almost always complex and multifactorial. Progress is routinely a product of trial and error. In more complex cases, patients take six months or even longer to establish a sustainable plan that works and is safe. When the plan is not working, it needs to be changed.

Patients with pain issues are commonly told there is nothing more that can be done for their pain. This is not true. I have found it possible to help patients safely and dramatically without ever being sure of the "why" for their pain. Results can be dramatic by simply focusing on helping their brains work better.

Patients do not always respond to standard measures. As a result, a physician may conclude that these patients cannot be helped through their services. This is different than concluding there is nothing more that can be done to better manage the patient's pain. The brain and central nervous system are highly adaptable. The brain is very capable of change and learning, arguably until it has deteriorated irreversibly as in end-stage dementia.

Some patients could benefit from more intense therapy such as prolonged inpatient care. Even when intense care may be indicated, patients and third-party payers commonly balk. Unfortunately, financial constraints frequently limit access to helpful interventions.

Family and psychological pressures also impede progress. Based on a patient's past experiences with prescribers and authority figures, a physician, particularly one who is a prescriber, may struggle to establish a therapeutic relationship. When patients do not like their physician or feel worse as a result of ongoing office visits, common sense indicates something is wrong.

Appropriate expectations in pain management is important and bears repeating. Using our pain scale, if a patient's pain levels are in the twenties or below out of the maximum score of 100, this reflects good pain management. Higher scores are quite acceptable for some, and one day a patient's pain score could be zero. Being pain free, however, is not a reasonable expectation for most complex pain patients. For some, almost miraculously, it does happen.

Treating chronic pain is similar to treating most chronic and relapsing diseases. If one seeks perfection in treating diabetics, one is likely to fail, become disappointed, or even cause harm. On the other hand, if one sees progress and ongoing reasonable blood sugar levels, outcomes are most favorable. Chronic pain management is similar, where progress and reasonable pain scores become indicators of good long term outcomes.

In life, things change. If a plan does not seem to be working as expected, adjustments are in order. When the plan is working, one may consider dropping some of the components of the plan to see what happens. No single recipe works for everyone. Options for patients are to be provided whenever reasonable or possible. Handouts and links related to pain management options may be helpful for some.

I suggest the options be considered similar to those on a menu at a restaurant. We choose from the myriad of options and see what works to help patients function better and feel better. If a patient wants help or suggestions in prioritizing what to try next, professional guidance can be most helpful. Over time through getting to know a patient an astute clinician can become confident that one option will likely work better than another. Nonetheless, both clinicians and patients are often humbled though the process of finding out what works.

Given the uncertainties in initial plans, it makes sense to start with the safest remedies and proceed from there. During the process of coming up with an effective plan, some of the slogans found in 12-step recovery programs can also be helpful. For example: "It takes time," "Progress, not perfection," "Easy does it," "Keep coming back," "It works if you work it," "It's a *we* thing," and "Take what's of use and leave the rest, these are but suggestions." Also, as in the care of substance use disorders, family therapy is often a helpful adjunct. Family members, even in their desire to be helpful, can make pain worse.

Chapter Three — What to Do When the Plan Is Not Working?

Chapter Three — What to Do When the Plan Is Not Working?

In summary:

1. The First Step Is Often to Make a Visit With One's Primary Care Provider.

2. The Next Step Is to Help Your Doctor Come Up With a Plan.

3. 10–Step "To Do" List to Help Your Doctor Help You

Despite adequate medical coverage, patients and caregivers are spending valuable time and effort to obtain medically indicated services. Often more than 50% of clinical time may be spent in debriefing and helping patients regarding third-party and regulatory issues.

Another common concern is limited access to proven effective medical care. Former pain clinics, which helped many patients, are simply no longer around. Third-parties will no longer pay for them. They are considered too expensive.

No quick resolution is forthcoming to counter the waste of time and resources related to regulatory and third-party involvement in medical care. In specialize pain management and addiction services administrative and regulatory concerns have become more of a problem than a help. The burdens they put on cost-effective medical care are enormous and widespread. Access to COAT in small towns and rural areas in the State of Washington has been limited further by recent legislation that has specific rules and regulations regarding the prescribing of opioids. Well-trained physicians often poorly understand the rules. Understandably colleagues have concerns because there is little in the way of legal precedent as to how the rules will be interpreted and enforced.

The liabilities have prompted several group practices to announce they will not provide opioids for chronic, non-cancerous pain. The liabilities are coupled with other factors that explain limited access to care: chronic pain management is inadequately reimbursed; many physicians are not prepared to safely and effectively manage chronic, complex pain with or without opioids; complex pain is often complicated by other medical concerns, such as substance use disorders, and other significant medical and mental health conditions; and, lastly, a team-oriented, collaborative approach to care is indicated. Given all these barriers to proper care, what can one do?

When confronting significant "system" problems over which we have little control, the best strategy is focusing on solutions and to come back to what we *can* do. The following is a list of suggestions and steps provided to help patients and their advocates stay focused on solutions.

1. Generally, the First Step Is to Schedule a Visit With One's Primary Care Provider.

See what your primary care provider will do for you. They are the medical practitioners who help patients receive necessary specialized care. Often in order to see a specialist, a proper referral is needed by a primary care provider. The following are some suggestions regarding a pain patient's dialogue with a primary care provider:

a. When a medical professional suggests a change in your medical regimen, ask on what basis or outcome will the change be judged? What is the time frame? How frequently will you be seen to assure progress? What assurance do they give if therapies prescribed are not adequate or if there are complications? What can or will be tried to provide at least a similar relief as that of your current regimen? Formally document the content of the conversation to better assure accountability. Physicians do forget what they said or agreed to and these sort of discussions tend not to be included in the medical record. Indeed, assure that the conversation is part of the medical record. When one finds that a medical record is in error or incomplete, patients have the right to have it corrected.

b. If one has an Opioid Use Disorder (OUD), be sure to explicitly discuss that. Even the Washington State pain rules confirm the importance of agonist therapy for patients with OUDs. [21] To not have access to proper agonist therapy provides a patient redress under the pain rules and formal professional standards.

c. Any physician at times must make recommendations that a patient doesn't like to hear, or is reticent about, whether it concerns prognosis, medications, surgery, hospitalization, behavioral therapy, diagnostic testing, stopping smoking, etc. The physician's professional responsibility is to assure that, if at all possible, long-term health improves as a result of referrals and other recommendations, let alone when they prescribe. Medical recommendations are best when based on individual needs in conjunction with available population and group-based studies (evidence-based medicine).

d. Primary care providers, or other physicians, are suppose to do more than simply inform you that they can't help you. All licensed practitioners have the responsibility to advocate for and help a patient obtain the best medical care. As already discussed, there are limits as to what any medical professional can provide. While someone may benefit from surgery, any good surgeon will not initiate therapy unless the means and follow-up are available to allow a healthy outcome. Let us limit energy spent in being critical or blaming. Focus on possible solutions first for you, then loved ones, and then for the greater community.

e. When patient harm or financial loss happens as a result of either a physician's failure to make an appropriate diagnosis or to not assure appropriate care, malpractice laws may apply. This is to be the last resort, because ultimately the process of malpractice litigation does not prevent patients from suffering, experiencing undue disability, or even dying. The process of a malpractice suit is also very stressful. This is not a prescription for well-being for anyone, let alone a patient with complex, chronic pain, or their family.

f. The Washington State's Medical Quality Assurance Commission is the governmental authority that oversees whether patients receive professional care from licensed practitioners. The commission can be contacted online and the office has a handout [22] on seeking advocacy/accountability through the commission.

2. How to Help Your Doctor Come Up With an Effective Plan for Your Pain Management.

The suggestions provided herein were tailored based on clinical experience in caring for patients living in Washington State's North Olympic Peninsula. Many patients here, as in other places, have struggled to find a physician who will prescribe them pain medications or agonist therapy for pain or opioid use disorders. The suggestions for these "local" patients may be used in conjunction with our List of Providers and our Letter to Colleagues. Other pertinent handouts are available online at www.OPAS.us.

No single recommendation will help every patient with every doctor. As with the best of medical care, individualized care is warranted. Nonetheless, certain principles and suggestions may help.

For a host of reasons, physicians may not feel comfortable prescribing controlled substances to patients. Your job is not to convince your physician to feel differently or to convince him or her of anything. Rather, attempt to better listen and understand the reasons they have for making their recommendations. If it is challenging to understand, it may not simply be your inability to understand medical explanations, but it could be a product of a dysfunctional health care system to which physicians fall victims as well.

In medicine there have always been different opinions about what constitutes the best care for a given patient. Decisions are sometimes based on "cultural" factors as much as scientific evidence or clinical expertise. Try not to focus just on what you think is needed, but continue to express a desire to receive the best of medical care. Understand that even the experts, such as those who promoted guidelines at the Center for Disease Control (CDC), can make guidelines under the influence of political and cultural factors, rather than simply on the current evidence, reasonable appraisals, and established effective approaches that limit medication-related complications.

10-Step "To Do" List to Help Your Doctor Help You

1. Make an Appointment.

2. Prepare for Your Visit.

3. Make Clear What You Want.

4. Work With Your Doctor.

5. Ask Questions.

6. Be Willing to Make Regular Visits

7. Educate Yourself.

8. Be Knowledgeable.

9. Ask for Referral.

10. Seek Mental Health care.

1. Make an Appointment.

In general, make an appointment at the office of a primary care provider, one you have been seen by within the previous three years. You are then by definition "an established patient." Make an initial appointment for a general checkup. Primary care providers are most inclined to investigate one's general medical care, rather than just addressing pain or addiction problems. If you do not have a primary care provider, it is time to take steps to get one. Your insurance provider should be able to give you a list of physicians who are accepting new patients in your area. Unless you are financially independent, or there are "concierge" physicians in your area, it is best to obtain some third-party coverage. When one's medical condition warrants consideration for ongoing opioids, third-party coverage is recommended.

2. Prepare for Your Visit.

Once with the doctor or primary care provider (PCP), and after customary introductions, you may acknowledge that you are anxious. You might also ask the clinician if you may record the conversation to help better process what you are told. Another option is to bring a friend or family member with you who will help record what is said and likely allay some of your anxiety. People do not function at their best when overly anxious.

It is advisable to review your medical record afterwards to make sure the discussions were properly and adequately recorded. One can always ask for corrections to the record when deemed appropriate.

Bring in old medical records you have which document who prescribed what and for what reasons. At the very least, it is helpful to bring in old prescription bottles. It is even better to bring in all the medications currently being prescribed to you. Doctors often now have access online to your list of currently prescribed controlled substances, but nothing helps more than seeing the actual prescription bottles.

3. Make Clear What You Want.

As much as possible, be as direct as you can in letting the doctor know what you want. You might find it helpful to express something like this: "Doctor, whether you have additional or better suggestions for my pain management, I would feel less anxious if I could have my prescriptions filled at their current level, at least until other options are on board and working. In my experience, it is my current regimen that works best. If we can find other safer, better options, I will be thankful. Of course, I am not happy about being dependent on these medications."

An alternative dialogue might start with "Doctor, I am very anxious about going through withdrawal and having worse pain. What are you specifically recommending I can do to help me avoid withdrawal symptoms and to more effectively manage my pain?"

If you haven't been formally evaluated for having an opioid use disorder, and there is a question about that, ask for such an evaluation. The criteria for an opioid use disorder are listed online and in reference[8]. Also, please review *Appendix One* to review the RODS screening tool. If you possibly have an opioid use disorder (OUD) inform your primary care provider of such.

Lastly, let him or her know that whenever possible or feasible, you intend to follow through as best you can with their professional recommendations.

4. Work With Your Doctor.

If the doctor indicates a need for more records or more diagnostic tests before he or she would feel comfortable prescribing you opioids or making changes to your regimen, acknowledge the request and your willingness to comply. This being said, do not hesitate to request further clarifications: "Doctor, my understanding is that complex, chronic pain cannot be readily measured by standard diagnostic tests, and these tests generally only provide clues as to why I might be in pain. How are the diagnostic tests you are ordering going to determine how much pain I am in or how much pain medications or other interventions I require for better pain management?" Alternatively, one might say: "Doctor, I am happy to complete any formal pain questionnaire, for I understand they are helpful to you and for me to assess my progress. How do you suggest we are able to go forward with my pain management? If you think it would be helpful, I am willing to see a pain specialist to validate my pain levels and plans for managing them."

Sometimes a doctor simply needs to confirm your prescriptions and assure you are not getting multiple prescriptions from multiple providers. This is reasonable. Fortunately, with the Washington State prescription monitoring program, a physician can now check that out while you are in the office.

When appropriate, thank your physician for helping you find other options besides pain pills to get relief for pain. Pills have limited results. Meanwhile, request that your pain be effectively addressed and remind them you want help to avoid any symptoms of withdrawal. Let them know that you are prepared to come back as often as they find necessary to help make sure that the medications are helping. You want any prescriptions to be part of a solution rather than a problem.

5. Ask Questions.

If they recommend lowering your dosage, ask them why. Ask them what they will do if the pain gets worse, or if you develop classic symptoms of withdrawal or suffer from other stress-related disorders. If they do not offer effective care for symptoms of withdrawal, ask them why not?

6. Be Willing.

Remember that our current payment system does not reward physicians for spending much time with a patient. Be willing to come back frequently to have your questions answered or to express your concerns. Let them know you are willing to attempt behavioral and other interventions. Access to the other possibly effective interventions need to be demonstrated. Often third-parties will not pay for much other than prescriptions, physical therapy, or common surgical procedures. If not yet tried, express a willingness to be tapered off of opioids with reassurance that available therapy will be as effective and safe as your current regimen. Ideally, the provision of the alternative therapy can be initiated prior to tapering, and when helpful can lead to a gentle tapering of opioids.

7. Educate Yourself.

If your physician brings up the new Washington State law as the reason they cannot prescribe, inform them that you have read it [21]. Share with the doctor that you do not see where the law prohibits them from maintaining patients on their current levels of opiates and that the rules state that prognosis is poor without agonist therapy (opioids) in patients with moderate or severe opioid use disorders. If they request a formal pain management consultation, agree to have one as soon as they can arrange it. Meanwhile, request that they prescribe adequate opioids for pain management to avoid any unnecessary withdrawal symptoms or worse pain management. Accept that any change in one's regimen, even very helpful ones, can initially aggravate pain. This is because any change promotes anxiety and anxiety can aggravate pain levels.

8. Be Knowledgeable.

If a doctor expresses that clinic or hospital policies do not allow them to prescribe you opioids or higher doses of opioids, then ask to see a copy of those policies. While confrontational, you might also ask whether those policies protect them from the legal and professional mandate to provide proper medical care.

If they recommend treatment for substance use disorders or other mental health conditions, ask them where you might get that help and ask for a formal referral. If you have or possibly have a substance use disorder and your physician recommends a state-licensed facility, other than a methadone clinic, remind them that agonist therapy and comprehensive medical care is not routinely available through state facilities. Inform them that state-licensed facilities rarely provide medical care. These facilities are also ill prepared to address chronic and complex pain.

Agonist therapy is often required for proper brain function in patients who have an OUD. If this seems to be news to them, provide them with references from the "Agonist" paper[10].

9. Ask for Referral.

If the doctor acknowledges feeling unqualified to manage your pain or addiction needs, thank the doctor for being forthright. Then ask them for a timely referral and, on account of your current medication regimen, if possible have the consultation set up before you leave.

Another option is for you to ask them, as noted above, if they are willing to work with a specialist to assure you receive the medical care required. Your primary care provider is responsible to help you obtain the best medical care, especially when that care could be life-saving. If he or she does not know who to call for help or where to send you, acknowledge the lack of expertise or access to same in the area. Offer to go out of the area when needed. Even Washington State's Medicaid program is required to transport patients out of an area to have access to necessary medical care.

Lastly, you might ask whether they feel comfortable stabilizing you medically until more specialized care is available. If they do not think it is medically indicated to limit symptoms of withdrawal or to adequately treat pain, then consider establishing medical care elsewhere and consider reporting them to the Medical Quality Assurance Commission.

The above may be the best option particularly if you feel they have qualified you simply as a "drug seeker." Prejudices and stigma exist toward patients on chronic opioids. Be prepared to get second opinions and, when indicated, inform the Medical Quality Assurance Commission of poorly managed pain or substance use disorders.[22] When a clinician writes off your symptoms as "drug seeking behavior" without an appropriate evaluation, this is unprofessional conduct and the consequences can be life-threatening. Drug seeking behavior is not a diagnosis! Patients have died or nearly died as a result of such medical care.

10. Seek Mental Health Care.

Any change to care, particularly care perceived to be helping and part of a long-term approach, is stressful for a patient. I advise all patients, who are struggling to get proper medical care, to seek out professional mental health services. Anxiety does not help pain or help the brain function better. Anxiety is a strong trigger for pain to flare up and to use substances inappropriately. At the time of your visit, you may also request a referral to a mental health professional, as well as to a pain or addiction specialist as needed. In general, obtaining optimal care for chronic pain management warrants one has advocates.

Afterward

Once we have assured care for ourselves or loved one, we all must wonder what we might do politically and socially to address the social concerns about access to necessary pain management care and the proper use of opioids. The over reliance on opioids for pain management has contributed to the current opioid abuse epidemic. It is nonetheless misguided to think that overprescribing is the root of the problem. The causes are quite complex. There are many political and cultural influences at play that influence the way one cares for patients with chronic pain and substance abuse disorders. These same factors even can influence the way that research is conducted and interpreted.

An example of potential cultural or political influences is the Center for Disease Control's emphasis on the lack of evidence of efficacy for opioids in pain management after 52 weeks. A recent review of the literature revealed that no medication which is prescribed for chronic painful conditions has demonstrated evidence for long-term efficacy. To single out opioids as lacking evidence for long-term efficacy appears to reflect prejudices regarding opioid prescriptions. All medications have known risks and all of them used in chronic painful conditions lack evidence for long-term efficacy. Furthermore, the benefits of opioids as demonstrated in clinical trials, are similar and sometimes superior to other medications. Granted, the improvements with opioids are generally marginal and in the twenty to thirty percent range for the populations studied. But, as with most FDA approved medications, there is a subset of patients who respond quite favorably to opioids and another subset poorly. Most research simply quantifies the "average" response to any given medication for any given indication. To single out opioids as lacking long-term efficacy as justification for limiting their use in chronic pain, while not acknowledging the widespread lack of such evidence for most medications and most procedures reflects cultural if not political influences.

The reader can review more of the author's thoughts and opinions on the current opioid epidemic in a small compendium entitled 'Opidemic' [23]. In addition, one can refer to the online publication regarding the cultural influences that contribute to substance abuse issues [24].

References / Resources

References / Resources

Clickable Links to online sources can be found in the online version of this book at DrRotchford.com/guide

1. "Syllabus Regarding the Basics of Chronic Pain and Its Management" [http://bit.ly/2EkpPVh] by J.K. Rotchford, M.D. 2003

2. "Chronic Pain Syndrome" [http://bit.ly/2EkpPVh] by Murray J. McAllister, PsyD

3. "Mystery of Chronic Pain," [http://bit.ly/2DX2nzM] a Ted Talk by Dr. Krane; reviews the evidence for considering chronic, non cancer pain a disease unto itself.

4. Interaction of pain, anxiety, mood disorders, sleep, and all the other variables that contribute to feelings. [http://bit.ly/2niEVTQ] J.K. Rotchford, M.D. 2017.

5. "Neuropathy" [http://bit.ly/2niLYfm] by J.K. Rotchford, M.D. (2016)

6. "The OPAS Experience," an [http://bit.ly/2nmeewY] an article in the journal the Pain Practitioner (Journal of the American Academy of Integrative Pain Management) by J.K. Rotchford, M.D. 2007.

7. "An Informal Review of Opioid Dependence (Addiction) Associated with Chronic Opioid Analgesic Therapy (COAT) for Chronic Pain" by [http://bit.ly/2GtD2fi] by J.K. Rotchford, M.D. (Title page only in Czech). Journal ADIKTOLOGIE 15(3) 2015.

8. Opioid Use Disorder—Diagnostic Criteria DSM-5 [http://bit.ly/2nq0qld]

9. "Role of maintenance treatment in opioid dependence" [http://bit.ly/2nq0qld] Ward J, et al.; Lancet 1999; 353:221-26.

10. "Agonist Therapy for Opioid Use Disorders" [http://bit.ly/2DL3ZNP] by J.K. Rotchford, M.D. 2016

11. "The Wrong Way to Treat Opioid Addiction" [http://nyti.ms/2Ei9Uqs] by Maia Szakvitzjan; New York Times Jan. 17, 2018.

12. "Brain Health 101" [http://bit.ly/2FpB5PE] by J.K. Rotchford, M.D., 2016

13. Addressing Anger associated with Addictions, and other Disabling Medical Conditions [http://bit.ly/2nfYtIM] by J.K. Rotchford, M.D., 2003

14. "Grief and the Grieving Process" [http://bit.ly/2nn0zFT] by J.K. Rotchford, M.D. (2016)

15. "Anxiety-a Discussion" [http://bit.ly/2DXG8cK] by J.K. Rotchford, M.D. Using anxiety as an example, a very brief review of the role of diagnoses, scientific methodology, and cultural factors and how they influence our therapeutic options. 2016.

16. "Four Simple Things to do to Eliminate Anxiety," [http://bit.ly/2nprX6i] Amen Clinic.

17. "Calming Trauma—How Understanding the Brain Can Help," [http://bit.ly/2GrMvU4] Dawn McClelland, PhD., Burn Support News, Fall 2008. p12-13.

18. "PTSD—A Primer For Patients" [http://bit.ly/2DWl1Ym] by J.K. Rotchford, M.D. 2016.

19. "Dealing With the Effects of Trauma," [http://bit.ly/2El0ASW] a great resource for lists of behavioral ways to more effectively reduce anxiety and feel safer. The publication was funded by the U.S. Department of Health and Human Services (DHHS), Substance Abuse and Mental Health Services Administration (SAMHSA), Center for Mental Health Services (CMHS), and prepared by Mary Ellen Copeland, M.S., M.A., under contract number 99M005957.

20. "Ketamine and Low Dose Therapy for Pain, Depression, and PTSD" [http://bit.ly/2El13EG] by J. K. Rotchford, M.D. 2015.

21. "Washington State Guideline on Prescribing Opioids for Pain" [http://bit.ly/2nhHAxc](2015 revised).

22. "Complaining to the Medical Commission" [http://bit.ly/2np26em] by J.K. Rotchford, M.D. 2017

23. Opidemic - Mapping our Way through the Opioid Crisis, [www.Opidemic.help] by J.K. Rotchford, M.D. 2017

24. "Cultural Factors within the United States Promote Substance Use Disorders: A Helpful Perspective for Responding to the Opioid Misuse Epidemic" [http://bit.ly/2FpD4U6] by J.K. Rotchford; MOJ Addiction Medicine and Therapy, Volume 4 Issue 1 - 2017

Appendices

Appendix 1

Rapid Opioid Dependence Screen (RODS)

Instructions: [Interviewer reads] The following questions are about your prior use of drugs. For each question, please indicate "yes" or "no" as it applies to drug use during the last 12 months or any 12 months..

1. Have you ever taken any of the following drugs?

    a.   Heroin   Yes ☐
        No ☐

    b.   Methadone   Yes ☐
        No ☐

    c.   Buprenorphine   Yes ☐
        No ☐

    d.   Morphine   Yes ☐
        No ☐

    e.   Other opioid analgesics   Yes ☐
        No ☐

(Eg: Vicodin, Darvocet, fentanyl, tramadol, hydrocodone, codeine, etc.)

If "Yes" answer questions 2-8.

2. Did you ever have to use more opioids to get the same high as when you started to use opioids?   Yes ☐ No ☐

3. Did the idea of missing a dose ever make you anxious? Yes ☐ No ☐

4. In the morning did you ever have to take a dose to avoid feeling dope sick or did you ever feel dope sick?   Yes ☐ No ☐

5. Did you worry about your use of opioids?   Yes ☐ No ☐

6. Did you ever find it difficult to stop or not use opioids? Yes ☐ No ☐

7. Did you ever have to spend a lot of time/energy obtaining opioids or recovering from feeling high or other effects?   Yes ☐ No ☐

8. Did you ever miss important things like dr.'s appointments, family/friend activities, or other things because of opioids?   Yes ☐ No ☐

Scoring: If 3 or more of questions 2-8 are "Yes," this is consistent with opioid dependence.

Appendix 2

Global Pain Scale

Instructions: For each question, please indicate your level of pain by circling a number from 0 to 10.

YOUR PAIN:

1. My current pain is:

No pain: 0 1 2 3 4 5 6 7 8 9 10 :Extreme pain

2. During the past week, the best my pain has been:

No pain: 0 1 2 3 4 5 6 7 8 9 10 :Extreme pain

3. During the past week, the worst my pain was:

No pain: 0 1 2 3 4 5 6 7 8 9 10 :Extreme pain

4. During the past week, my average pain was:

No pain: 0 1 2 3 4 5 6 7 8 9 10 :Extreme pain

5. During the past 3 months, my average pain was

No pain: 0 1 2 3 4 5 6 7 8 9 10 :Extreme pain

YOUR ACTIVITIES: *during the past week I was NOT able to:*

6. Go to the store ....

Strongly Disagree: 0 1 2 3 4 5 6 7 8 9 10 :Strongly Agree

7. Do chores in my home ....

Strongly Disagree: 0 1 2 3 4 5 6 7 8 9 10 :Strongly Agree

8. Enjoy my friends and family

Strongly Disagree: 0 1 2 3 4 5 6 7 8 9 10 :Strongly Agree

9. Exercise (including walking)

Strongly Disagree: 0 1 2 3 4 5 6 7 8 9 10 :Strongly Agree

10. Participate in my favorite hobbies or perform normal tasks:

Strongly Disagree: 0 1 2 3 4 5 6 7 8 9 10 :Strongly Agree

YOUR FEELINGS: *during the past week I have felt:*

11. Afraid   Strongly Disagree: 0 1 2 3 4 5 6 7 8 9 10 :Strongly Agree

12. Depressed   Strongly Disagree: 0 1 2 3 4 5 6 7 8 9 10 :Strongly Agree

13. Tired   Strongly Disagree: 0 1 2 3 4 5 6 7 8 9 10 :Strongly Agree

14. Anxious   Strongly Disagree: 0 1 2 3 4 5 6 7 8 9 10 :Strongly Agree

15. Stressed   Strongly Disagree: 0 1 2 3 4 5 6 7 8 9 10 :Strongly Agree

YOUR CLINICAL OUTCOMES: *during the past week:*

16. I had trouble sleeping
          Strongly Disagree: 0 1 2 3 4 5 6 7 8 9 10 :Strongly Agree
17. I had trouble feeling comfortable
          Strongly Disagree: 0 1 2 3 4 5 6 7 8 9 10 :Strongly Agree
18. I was less independent
          Strongly Disagree: 0 1 2 3 4 5 6 7 8 9 10 :Strongly Agree
19. Unable to work or take on normal responsibilities
          Strongly Disagree: 0 1 2 3 4 5 6 7 8 9 10 :Strongly Agree
20. I needed to take more medicines
          Strongly Disagree: 0 1 2 3 4 5 6 7 8 9 10 :Strongly Agree

Total Score: _____

Add the ***total score and divide by 2.*** Each subset is worth 25 points. The maximum total score is 100.

Your score: _____

Basic OPAS Follow-Up Office Questionnaire:

Intended for: Patients with chronic pain, substance use disorders, or with any diagnosis or medication use related to brain health.

Instructions: Since your last visit, **please circle** any of the following symptoms you have had: constipation, diarrhea, nausea, anorexia, weight loss or gain, malaise/fatigue, problems with concentration, memory problems, irritability, hopelessness, anxiety, legal problems, loss of feeling or strength, thoughts of hurting yourself/suicide. For each question the **lower** the score **the better** you are.

Other possible concerns?_____

1. How have your relationships with significant others or immediate family members been during the past month?

    0 1 2 3 4 5 6 7 8 9 10   ____

Delightful and wonderful relations – Nobody wants to be around me

2. Please rate your fear of financial insecurity during this past month.

    0 1 2 3 4 5 6 7 8 9 10   ____

No fear of financial insecurity – Fear of starvation or dying from exposure

3. How far along are you in meeting your goals of pain relief, recovery, or general well-being?

    0 1 2 3 4 5 6 7 8 9 10   ____

I've met all my goals – It's all hopeless

4. How many legal worries have you had during the past three months?

    0 1 2 3 4 5 6 7 8 9 10   ____

None – In jail the whole time

5. How happy with your living situation have you been during the past month?

0 1 2 3 4 5 6 7 8 9 10   ____

Couldn't be better – Couldn't be worse

6. During last week how much time have you spent in thinking about or seeking pain relief, medications, alcohol, or drugs of abuse?

0 1 2 3 4 5 6 7 8 9 10   ____

None – Every awake minute

7. How abstinent from non-prescribed, mind-altering substances have you been during the past month?

0 1 2 3 4 5 6 7 8 9 10   ____

Total Abstinence – Daily Relapse of all drugs/alcohol

8. How would you rate your overall physical health?

0 1 2 3 4 5 6 7 8 9 10   ____

Superb – Expect death in next week

9. How would you rate your overall mental/emotional health?

0 1 2 3 4 5 6 7 8 9 10   ____

As well as can be imagined – As bad as can be imagined

10. How would you rate your overall spiritual health?

0 1 2 3 4 5 6 7 8 9 10   ____

Feel loving Higher Power is in charge – Feel totally alone and hopeless

Total Score   _____

Appendix 3

OPAS Behavioral Plan Discussion

Patients with chronic, complex pain, substance use disorders, or other conditions which benefit from a healthy brain are often helped by "behavioral" changes. To help appreciate the interplay between standard medical/surgical interventions and "behavioral" interventions, the metaphor of the brain being like a computer is useful. The brain gets input, processes the input, and then produces an output similar to a computer. In computers the hardware and software, while integrated, do not change one another. If a computer is malfunctioning, one must wonder if it is a hardware problem, software problem, or both. In the case of the brain, however, the brain's software can transform brain hardware (structural and physiological findings). Likewise, the brain's hardware problems can change the software programming. Therefore, the brain's software and hardware are not only integrated, but they can change each other.

Some examples might help. Patients who are prescribed antidepressants after a time will start to behave differently and think differently about a whole host of things, even their belief in God can change. The opposite is also true! When one changes one's thinking and behavior, one may change the actual structure of the brain! Even with a serious degenerative disease such as dementia, "exercising" the brain, through certain "behavioral" efforts, potentially reverses some of the structural changes. Doing yoga regularly, for example, has been shown scientifically to increase "grey matter," the important responding, organizing, remembering, and executive components of the brain. Bottom line, behavioral interventions can help the brain function better and, over time, may even change the structure as well as the chemistry of the brain.

The potential for behavioral interventions to improve brain function are enormous. In turn, healthier brains promote better pain management, recovery from addictions, reduced anxiety, improved immune function, better relationships, and often promote progress with other medical issues such as heart or breathing problems.

A challenge is to find the best behavioral plan for each person. Given the variations in "software," let alone "hardware," in our different brains, it makes sense that plans are best individualized. Because there are often limited clinical trials to guide us, a trial and error approach is commonly used. As a physician, my job is to help patients establish plans that make sense and are likely to help. Nonetheless, it often comes down to a trial and error effort. A team effort, though, is often essential!.

While one's plan is likely to change with time, it is important to have one. Formal plans help to evaluate, over time, what might or might not be working.

Making a Plan

When starting to establish a treatment plan, a factor to remember is that multiple combined interventions often work best. Of course, it makes sense to start with the safe, easy, and readily available options. When there are proven effective interventions for your condition, we plan to implement those first. If, however, one limits interventions to ones that are "proven efficacious," outcomes are often compromised.

In establishing your plan for better brain health, another principle is, from the first, to emphasize changes that promote better homeostasis. Homeostasis is just a fancy way of helping to maintain stability and balance. The brain doesn't do well with "ups and downs," and we want to do what we can to promote more "regular" functioning of the brain.

For example, when long-acting medicines are prescribed to be taken routinely, at the same time every day, better brain homeostasis is promoted. When brains are in a better state of homeostasis, we are safer, and we often feel safer. Any intervention which promotes a greater state and sense of "safety" is likely to help brains work better. That being said, differences between people regarding what promotes safety are common and comprise one reason why plans are best individualized to see what works best.

Lastly, any plan for change can by itself create anxiety. Change threatens the "status quo." So, all good plans for significant change must include support and structure, particularly early on in the process. In many patients it helps when the changes occur slowly over time.

Your Plan as of _____/_____/_____

Passive Elements of Your Plan: (things being done to you or for you; for example: medications, procedures, testing, doctor visits, therapy, etc.)

1. _____
2. _____
3. _____
4. _____
5. _____

Active elements of your plan: things you are doing differently; for example changes in diet, exercise, daily routines, relationships, and living changes such as work, pleasure, spiritual, or religious practices, taking medications as directed, rather than as needed, studying about what works, etc.

1. _____
2. _____
3. _____
4. _____

5. _____

6. _____

7. _____

Note: attempt to have more active elements of your plan than passive ones. In the short run passive modalities are often effective, but the active changes are associated with the best long-term outcomes.

To help your healthcare team better care for you, we suggest you keep a folder of your current plans and keep a "diary" of what seems to work best for you. In my experience, patients rarely do this, but to update your plan after each visit makes sense. It all takes time, for the brain most often heals slowly over months and years, rather than over days or weeks.

Finally: list some of what you expect to change for the better as a result of your above plan. Keep the focus on positive things, rather than avoidance of negative ones:

_____

_____

_____

About the Author

J. Kimber Rotchford, M.D., M.P.H has longstanding expertise in treating outpatients who suffer from chronic pain, addictions, and related disorders. Dr. Rotchford is among the earliest pain management specialists, certified by the American Academy of Integrative Pain Management. Since 1981, he has emphasized and implemented integrative approaches to pain management.

His enduring interest and expertise in pain management led Dr. Rotchford to become a specialist in Addiction Medicine. He is one of the first physicians to be board certified in addiction medicine through the American Board of Addiction Medicine. He is the author of professional publications related to pain management and addiction medicine.

Dr. Rotchford is passionate about finding effective and practical solutions for pain management, as well as for the opioid crisis. He has a strong background in Public Health and is a longstanding Fellow of the American College of Preventive Medicine. A native of Washington, he is a graduate of the University of Washington's School of Medicine and School of Public Health. The University of Washington has a noteworthy history of leadership and expertise in both chronic pain management and Public Health. He has also studied, worked, and taught internationally.

Recognized for his compassion and his expertise in the treatment of chronic pain and opioid use disorders, Dr. Rotchford has practiced for his entire clinical career in small towns in Washington State. First, he served patients on Washington's Pacific coast. For the past 25 years he has practiced medicine in Port Townsend on the state's Olympic Peninsula.

Dr. Rotchford's full curriculum vitae is online at www.OPAS.us/resume

Acknowledgements: Dr. Rotchford wants to thank Ms. Andie Mitchell for her editing suggestions in recent revisions which complemented the professional services and encouragement of Mr. Dan Youra, without whom, this book would have never happened.

About the Editor

Dan Youra is an author, editor-in-chief, and publisher of books and magazines at Youra Media. He is chairman of the board of directors for a not-for-profit, medical clinic in Port Townsend, Washington.

A Sampling of Reviews of Dr. Rotchford

Dr. Rotchford's approaches are "cutting edge for addressing problematic opioid use in high-risk patients."

Alex Cahana, M.D., Chief, Division of Pain Medicine
University of Washington Medical Center

"Poster boy" for the cost effective, scientific, and successful treatment of pain and addiction patients."

Samuel W. Shoen, M.D.

"I've met several people who were under Dr. Rotchford's care, none of whom had a problem transitioning from narcotic treatment to being medication free."

Audrey L. Fain, Ph.D. (retired) Registered Nurse CA-WA

"Well regarded Pain Management consultant and has been recognized as a leader in the state."

Alan G. Greenwald, M.D., Orthopedic Surgeon

Other Publications by J. Kimber Rotchford, M.D.

Available online at www.DrRotchford.com under handouts tab

Addiction & Brain Health
What Promotes Recovery from Addictions
Brain Health 101
Help for Family Members
Trust—Making It a Non-Issue
PTSD—A Primer for Patients
Quitters Guide to Recovery from Marijuana and other Addictions
Self-Medicating
Medical Use of Addictive Substances

Pain Management
Review of Opiate Dependence in Pain Patients on Chronic
Opioid Agonist Therapy (COAT)
Syllabus – Basics of Chronic Pain and Its Management
"The OPAS Experience,"article in *Pain Practitioner*
Neuropathies—A Brief Overview
Managing Acute Pain in Patients on Buprenorphine
Managing Acute Pain in Patients Prescribed Methadone

Medications
Agonist Therapy—Buprenorphine and Methadone Therapy
Buprenorphine Patient Syllabus
Ketamine and Low Dose Therapy for Pain
Naltrexone to Treat Opiate Addiction
Probuphine—Game Changer for Opioid Use Disorders

Adjunctive Care
ACUPUNCTURE—A Brief Introduction
Medical Cannabis (Marijuana)—A Physician's Experience
Anxiety—A Discussion
Anger Issues in Those With Pain or Addiction Concerns
Grief and Grieving

Olympas Medical Services
J. Kimber Rotchford, M.D.

Olympas Pain and Addiction Services Clinic
1136 Water St. Suite 107
Port Townsend, WA 98368

www.OPAS.us
staff@OPAS.us

www.ingramcontent.com/pod-product-compliance
Lightning Source LLC
Chambersburg PA
CBHW081627220526
45468CB00009B/2328